THE PRIORY PRINCESS

Time Frozen

By
Jessica Button

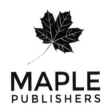

MAPLE
PUBLISHERS

The Priory Princess

Author: Jessica Button

Copyright © Jessica Button (2023)

First Published in 2023

ISBN 978-1-915796-33-2 (Hardback)

Book cover design and Book layout by:
    White Magic Studios
    www.whitemagicstudios.co.uk

Published by:
    Maple Publishers
    Fairbourne Drive, Atterbury,
    Milton Keynes,
    MK10 9RG, UK
    www.maplepublishers.com

A CIP catalogue record for this title is available from the British Library.

I dedicate this book to my mother who turned 78 this year. She is my most enthusiastic critic and loves my work. Mummy has suffered secondary lung cancer this year 2022 but she still defies all odds and is a remarkable example of positive energy and how this can transform one's life for the better. I also would like to take this opportunity to thank all the staff and lovely amazing women who work at Equinox, a charity set up for women's service. You all have helped make this book a reality for me so thank you from my heart.

CONTENTS

Introduction

My name is Jessica Button and I am a 34 year old women...

I currently reside in a charity scheme set up for vulnerable women called Equinox.

There are several places around the country of the unique scheme one in London I am currently residing in the one in Brighton.

My episodes and so forth started when I was 21 in particular when I was first diagnosed with schizophrenia I have since been told that I am schizo affective instead but it boarders along the same lines.

I'm not just my label though. So here's a bit about me! I am a professional drummer. I worked hard at this since age 15 and have played gigs all over Brighton, Tenerife and Devon. I went to The British Institute of Modern music. Drumming is the heart beat to my soul and helps me think and I become meditative whilst playing.

I found myself in the Priory Ticehurst in the summer and autumn of 2021, whereby the didn't have a drum kit, so, I started to write poetry to mediate. Having been well read with my first degree at Chichester University when I was 18 in English literature I felt the passion to write. The syllabic tone rhythm and vibe and Symantec's of each poem would mean a lot to me and I felt I could create a little space on page that utterly summed up my emotions.

I would bring a poem with me to read to the psychiatrist each weekly ward round, to which she always gently and politely replied "beautiful Jessica" you see this is where I discovered that my poems did not only just help me but they would and could help others to, with multiple meanings at each read. When it was my time to go the psychiatrist at the beautiful priory hospital Ticehurst asked me to write a poem about the ward and for it to be put up near the medicine clinic where all could read and hopefully be inspired to help them on their journey too, to get well.

I left a last legacy there and it was such an honour.

I am now in recovery but I still keep on writing about all topics that I can dream of or feel or even which happen to me.

This is a never ending journey and I hope you all will enjoy the ride with me!

I dedicate this book to my poorly mother suffering secondary lung cancer in her last remaining lung and I pray that the successes of my life can rejuvenate her spirits and help her to feel the positive vibes and keep her breathing for as long as is conceivable. Well of course, to infinity and beyond! Hospital.

Today was a big day

Yeah, you should listen to this

Jump right into the obis
Like it never happened

The gangs that wanted to murderer me
Seem to disappear like;
Light on a shadow

Well, what do ya know

Mummy is really unwell
She put on a brave face

That's how we are in this
Human race

Winners, we won't ever give up

I'll fight for my life
And she'll fight for hers

Amen

No time to die

Today is a new day
Maybe one of the toughest
So far,
So far away from where I want to be

It's so hard, not to be free
It's a fight, tonight
World war 3 on Jessica Bond
Who lost her Bond girl

Give it a swirl, have a go
See how far you'd actually go
Are you really going to murder me?
Really? You're that evil

Like the devil
I'm in hell
I saw the blood on my old phone
But guess what; I'm not alone

Let me live, back off
Back off, back off, back off
My life is precious to me
I'm not a thug like them

We have to be brave

Not a slave
To love to happiness to everything
That's just
Too good
To be true

I feel so scared still
But guess what with free will
I may make it out
Be free to go out n about

It's tough in here
Doesn't ease my fear

But if I got out
Would I only shout
Out loud I ain't proud

Of this terror
My own error

Re wire my brain
I don't think I'm insane

Maybe but I know what
I'm in pain

God it gets hard

Harder than I could have ever imagined

When the heart tells you one thing
But the brain's saying another
When I've learnt over the years into
To live my life, quite differently to others

I follow my heart

I guess it's how everyone recovers
And sees logic over lust

Sensibility over love
And responsibility over impulse

That's the way to be in this world

Fuck it fuck it fuck it

What's the point!?
Always alone
I haven't grown

Out of this mess
What a state
Is this girl
Called Jess

I don't know what to do
Fall in love again
Then what
My heart will be broken
I shouldn't have spoken

Even a fling
Something
Would be nice

Go with the flow
Don't stop the river
Allow it to be
And we shall see
I might feel finally free
And we'll all be, so happy!!

What a wonderful life

How to get past this god for stricken strife
Of Dis contempt

Look at me standing
Here on my own again

Does this work for you all
When my mental health
Takes the piss from who I would could be

When I'm a position in my own right to think
Yes I can breath in and out

The oxygen in the air, is there
For us all

In the mood to create

Get myself out of this state
Open my mind
Let's reiterate

Only to find a hollow
Nothing
Absolutely nothing

Can that be true
Is it me or is it you
Who grew

Out of this love
Forces from above
Can't save me now

Like sunshine on pale skin

It burns
When's it my turn
This ice I'm treading on is so thin

I'm so so so scared right now
Fingers crossed and that's all I can do
It's so painful

To be this person without a clue
I'm stuck in this colour blue
Ain't that true

Anyway what's the point
Without her I gotta keep going

Keep this life of mine flowing
Without knowing is hell

This is the longest half an hour of my life
Mummy I love you so much it hurts

Your the bravest lady in the world
Not many could have been so 100 per cent
Positive

The sun shines

Like chimes
The birds chirp

What you say?
Who's the jerk!
No one it's a mistake

Can we retake
This time again
Remember me ok

My lips stain
No lipstick fun today
Not for another decade my friend

Well maybe less
But I know I won't lend
My heart out again

All is well
There's no spell

What's that you say

Take away my rights
You must be out of your mind
Cos it's not Often you will find
The time to have peace in yourself
If they take away all that's mine

We hear the cries of the ladies of America
It's not fair or good to create this kind of
Hysteria

As women we can stand together
Who's says we have to do what men dictate
Sister hood is so much stronger

Weaken yourself to lend your rights away
No
You can't say
What we do with our bodies

Women should have the right to choose
Otherwise, it's just societies that will loose

More women.
Will die
Is that what you call a world that's flying high?!

The instruction of man to dictate to us
Will only make the destruction
Of human life

In the end you will see that it's not the way
Go and have a rethink cos us women that
are here to stay, say
These are our own bodies
And we will do whatever we want
Against whatever you say

Summer vibes

And I'm feeling fine
Magnums a plenty
What's that £20?! For that

Gosh the prices have gone up this year
But that won't get me down
There's no need to frown
When The sun is out I act like a clown

So to yet another day in this place
Don't mistake my smile for all is not a race
Just I like to smile once in a while
And there's nothing better than summer vibes

Bright lights big colours pumping music
Face paint and we're away!!
Skip jump put your hands up
As the crowds glees in excitement

I put my tunes on and it's like wow weee
I didn't know it was possible again

To feel so free

And that's all it was a DJ session
And the people can't get enough

Now ain't that a lesson
Stop the tears stop the fears
It's summer time baby
That's what I told this lady

So pride has come and gone
But it never ends here in Brighton
Let's get together and get that fight on
To help those around us and all that suffer

The wondrous world

Of the priory
Don't forget to write this in you diary

Each week we have a ward round
Then sometime our lost souls
Will be found

It's not an average life here
I know that having lived
In total fear

Screams and cries
Who do we trust
Is it all lies!?

In time we can see that with also
The help of meds and a warm bed
That we will live again and be
Discharged to go

Then it's up to us
To make our lives beautiful again
And not depend on others
This is how all recovers

What do we do tonight

When there's so much to do
And not so much light

Might I say
What do we do
With a broken radio
And a senseless tv

These things don't help me feel free
The monotonous trail
Of every day
Gets to me at times

I just miss those Devon days
When my life wasn't such a haze

Of despair and regret
I don't ever want to forget
You

Cos it's true what they say
Life flies when you're having fun
But it stops still when we lose the thrill

So, I say to you
Rise high up into the sky
And see the stars
It will help with all those broken
Hearts
And lost scars

Heroin

Is like
Resin for my wounds

It fills my system up
So that I can't even
Hiccup

It's what I need
As I bleed
My life away

What's that you say
Stop
Well pop yo are not here

Who could save me
As I shed a tear

It's not me it's them
The stress of being
So tough
Has got to me

Now I'm a junkie

And so

The story goes
She loves my mum
And like that
I just feel so dumb

I love mummy so much
And as such I'm pleased that
My friends all adore her

But sometimes it would be nice
If they loved me as much

Don't worry I no longer want your touch
But I've forgotten how to be free

And be happy
The grief and trauma stresses have somewhat
Made me
Not
Who I truly am

I can't be doing that badly tho
I'll just see where this road leads me
And go with the flow
Cos mother neither you nor I actually know

Where did it all go?

All the lovely Devon folk
The calm the peace
The beauty

Where did it all go?

When does my mind get a brake

From being in this state
I tell ya
It ain't
A holiday

I wish so much I could work
Work it all out
So that I can be free

Would you want that yourself
To live without fear
My dear
This is what I say

Fuck them!!!!!!

Is this going to be

The best thing I've ever fuckin written
Once shy twice bitten
Just give me a damn kitten

In all honesty
I don't know which way this is going to go

This ain't just for show
Mummy don't you know
I'm sure you jolly well do

The sun rises and it's a new dawn
For you and me love this life
To the max
Exactly that
Have you got a hat for that?

Thing is this story can't end
From every point of the world
I'll always defend you
I love you sooooooooooooo much
You're my everything

I can't carry on
With no parents that's not right
Surly?! God stop this now
Oh wow
What's that you won't listen

Well, I have news for you
Mummy will always be alive
Always glisten in my heart
Like the sea in a sunny day

This way she's always gonna
Stay
Alive

It's like some kind of paradise

That I find myself in
When I look at you
I begin; to think of the future
Cos you're a beaut yeah!

And I tread this path
Delicately
Remember me

Don't be a stranger
Reverse, rewind this time
Or let's do it again even better
With some wine

That would be Divine, if only
You were mined

Or as a friend, anything you can lend yourself to be.
Then I know that I will be happy

I don't pine for it anymore

I don't care what you think
In a blink
And I'm gone to the midst of time
With my wine
I feel just fine

Please don't enter my world again
I feel stronger inside
Against this divide
Of them and us
What's more that we
Could possibly need to discuss

I have no home
But I've grown
Older and fatter
Does it matter

I want to go home in my heart
I have a lump in. My throat
That we had to eventually part

This is all I've got
My soul my mind and
My art

Darling no words

Other than
I love you
The love of a mother
Can't be broken

The love reciprocated
Back
Can't be spoken

These three words
I love you

Come from the soul
The soil of the earth
The air we breath
Just believe

When you can see me
It's easier to feel it
When I can see you
It's easier too

Relax now Jessica
Go with the flow

Cos we can't always know
What tomorrow might bring
And guess what
It's nearly spring

Poor unfortunate souls

That end up here
We lost our roles
In life

Each day is agony
The monotony
Of the life in the house
But still
I can't go outside
All I can do is hide

If I abide, by the rules
Will I think more of myself
Your all god damn fools
To think I can cope

I can't
It's as simple as that
As I put on my next hat
For the big day
Skip a beat
And say hurray
Or cry in dismay

If I had a chance

I would change my life
If I had a chance
I would reverse the time
If I had a chance
I would sip less wine
I'd stand tall
I'd be fit and have kept
My beautiful, toned body
That matched my long blonde hair
And prettier face

If I had a chance
I would re write my story
So, we could all live
In this kinda glory

If I had a chance …..
what would you do,
If you had the chance?

I'd refuse the meds
So they could never have got
Into my head

Megan

I'm in heaven
The priory that is

Stick to the rules
I feel like I'm back
At my old schools

You caught me n Kate
Maybe that was our fate
Or were we just too late!

But really, you're a good lady
Funny and nice, you add spice
To otherwise, rubbish days.

Thanks Megan

Tonight is a night of reflection

Detection of the inspection
Of the spotless mind

You see they're hard to find
I wouldn't care
If it wasn't fair

But then again
We could be on
The mend

For this I must depend
On me

It makes me quite emotional to think

This building was here hundreds of years ago
In one second not even a blink

And I will be gone
Suffice to say
I didn't wanna stay

But I'll dearly miss
The days I had here
Living at times without so much fear

Am I truly healed
I think so
Onto my next mountain to climb
This thing called life

Go go go
I won't leave you behind.......

Don't forget about me

You are so beautiful to me
Your everything I hope for
Your everything I need

Anthony is my mate

He's really great

We get into debates about life;

Far too many people in this world
Cause aggro

But we are chilled man
So laid back

What a crack
He's great he's a warm soul

Oh well it's not the end
Don't pretend

I'll meet you in hove
And have a dose
On the beach
What a life
We lead

So happy I think I'll be
When we are all finally free

Whereas I did have the time

This seems to be what I chose

It's not
Take it back
Stop

I can't take it now
I couldn't take it before
It's like some kinda law

This diagnosis
That I suffer from
I'm gone

Out the door
Your more
Then I ever asked for

So, thanks
I'll take with me gratitude
It's just my
Kinda attitude

Sarah is delectable
She a right character
She so kind and nice

As a manger
Go her

I think sometimes
She may worry too much

But as such I can reassure

I'll be polite respectable at all
times
Even if my poems don't rhyme

What will be

Will be
What era were you born in?
Does it really matter
Cos we still all agree the same
Morning

It may seem quite boring
Don't question why she needs to be free
She will just say
It's the way to be

Loose your dreams
And you could lose your mind

Please if you will

Please let me feel you
Inside me is a pain
That you recovered
Now that, I found you
I recovered

But now you're gone
How can it be so simple
So hard horrible and pure
Are you sure

Can't we be friends
Or is this how it always ends

I miss you SO much

God give me hope
Please if you will
Let me feel you

I can feel your heartbeat now
In my mind
And it feels divine

Where did tenderness go

Soft to touch
One day we'll all wake up
And see that

If there was a 19-year-old philosopher
Who had all the answers
Would he be more or less mature
Then a 50 year old whose lived it
But still hasn't got a clue

To be in the middle is where I'm at
Finding my balance is key
That's what it is
To truly be happy

Justine

I mean
This is obscene

Imagine that
They hurt me
But then I flew
BIMM
Away so fast
It's all my past
Wouldn't last

Anyway, let's talk about you
Cos there ain't many
That really have a clue

Unlike you, Justine.

Here's a happy poem

For a genuine person

she is so beautiful
I can't explain

Her personality lights up her face
Her good heart is clear to see

That's the kinda lady she is
Calm cool collected

In the nicest possible way
I just wanted to say
I love you Kerry
You make us all so merry!

How is it that the worst times of your life end up

Being the best times?!
By which I mean having no job no kids no husband
no wife no life
Nothing
No responsibilities no one to love and be loved back
no home no career no money
I ain't got nothing
I hear ya
And yeah, in this homeless street drug alcohol mental
health charity I feel happy
Like I was in psychiatric

Sam hull
Is savvy and she ain't dull

So pretty is she
Makes everyone just and skip
So happily

She has an important role in the house
Deputy manager and all that

But Sam has a generous and kind approach
Maybe I shouldn't have spoke
Too soon!

No all will always be well when you know Sam
Cos she's the lady that can't ever
Go unnoticed

Bill as you will

Will, fill your world with colour
It didn't matter with bill
What state you are in

She will always have open arms
To catch you m
Never shall you fall
If you know bill

She such a good soul
Everybody needs
To know this
About our bill

Helen melon

Can be quite a challenge
Maybe hardest than all

To imagine her soft heart
She really worlds apart
For the average

Helen is a deeply caring lady
Don't be dismissed by her

She come and get ya
Only on the kindest way

Cos Helen only wants the best
For everyone

Tor I'm in awe

How to run such a slick project
When there's so many variables
You make managing this joint
Seem bearable

Thanks for for popping in
In the odd month from time to time

I can tell you how well I'm doing now
Cos of yours ladies
Equinox is a special place

Debbie well what can I say

You've been the best and always will be
Last summer you literally
Saved
My
Life

How you do it don't know
What just goes for show
Is that your a true professional
With the best interest of the
Service user at heart

I've had other workers but non seemed
To care so much
Maybe it's just your flare for this job

But my god, I can't thank you enough
You make them all seem so rough
Although you can be quite tough
On me

It's only for me to understand and see
The world that we live in

Im always forever thankful to you
Debbie

Janie

Well, what DO I say
She the manager
Let's all say one big hip hip hurray

I'm all seriousness she seems to be good
A lot more ordered
If you like that kinda thing?!

She was calm and composed
One day
When I was in a real state

I won't forget it
And now I think we can relate
A bit better

Thank you, Janie

Keren Dale

Isn't male
No! That's right she's a dancer
With the answer!

Who would have known it
This bright springy
Gorgeous lady

Can dance the town away.
With her Pizzazz
You'll never be down

She's always there
To spread the cheer
I love having Keran around

And as my key worker
I've fallen on my feet
No, I won't skip a beat!

What it means to be a women and what a women is

Questions we've been asking for 2000 years
Empowering each other
The suffrages and suffragettes let's not forget
Historically women have been treated as second to
men

And then again
We remember what the pioneers did for women,
lasting legacies that transformed
Our position in society
And the riots you see
We set ourselves free of all the constraints
With all our empowering debates

To be a woman is a multi-faceted thing
With wonders and treasures a plenty
Listen gents now you see

The figure of a lady has been adored throughout time
It's really rather Divine
All the shapes and sizes we can be

We born our children
We give and hold life inside us
That bursts to get out
It's truly incredible

Women can empower other women.
Choose to be kind and wise
And the world will see
There's no limits
To our delightful tree
Of life

Loopy Luna

Isn't so loopy
She's sassy and well she ain't
Trashy but she has a big brain

Intellectual actually
And quite a hidden depth

Luna is so cool
She didn't even mind the fools

I think Luna is one of a kind
Mind you so am I
Wonderful she is

A true gem in my heart

Fatima

Well, what can I say

If I may
Your cooking is divine
And if I had some time
I'd love to cook with you

You a mother of all
And a feeder to our empty stomachs

But this house is full of big hearts
Fatima, I thank you from the bottom
Of mine
For all the lovely food you create for
Us all

Tom ridge watch out

She ain't afraid to shout

A heart of gold is this lady
So true and wise but also fun

I can see myself sitting with Tom
And a gin n tonic

Actually, I hate that stuff
Oh, how ironic!

I do love Tom
She da bomb!

The subtle changes

The alchemy
Of repent

Makes me decent from what's real
In this one life it's easy to conceal

Who we really are how we feel
And then you see
We beg borrow or steel

It's not a surprise whilst in this
Rather static disguise

That I I end up in sodom and
gamora

Oh where did beauty go

www.ingramcontent.com/pod-product-compliance
Ingram Content Group UK Ltd.
Pitfield, Milton Keynes, MK11 3LW, UK
UKHW041302280225
4809UKWH00002B/11

9 781915 796332